The Self-Care Lighthouse: A Nurse's Guide To Weathering Life's Storms

Acknowledgment

I would like to express my heartfelt gratitude to those who supported me in bringing *The Self-Care Lighthouse: A Nurse's Guide to Weathering Life's Storms* to life.

First and foremost, I extend my deepest appreciation to my fellow nurses and healthcare professionals. Your resilience and dedication inspired the creation of this guide. Thank you for sharing your experiences, struggles, and triumphs, which served as a beacon of hope and guidance throughout this journey.

I am immensely grateful to my family and friends for their unwavering encouragement and support. Your belief in my vision helped me navigate the challenges I faced while writing this book. To my partner, thank you for your patience and understanding during those late nights and early mornings when I was lost in thought, pen in hand.

Special thanks to my mentors and colleagues who provided invaluable insights and feedback. Your expertise and encouragement pushed me to refine my ideas and ensure that this guide resonates with those seeking solace and strength.

Finally, I would like to acknowledge the countless individuals who have shared their stories of resilience and self-care with me. Your courage in weathering life's storms inspired me to create a resource that I hope will empower others to prioritize their well-being.

This book is a tribute to the nursing community and a reminder that even in the most challenging times, we can find our way back to the light through self-care and support.

Dedication

To all the dedicated nurses and healthcare professionals who navigate the turbulent waters of care with compassion and resilience. Your strength in the face of adversity serves as a guiding light for others.

This book is dedicated to those who prioritize the well-being of others, often at the expense of their own self-care. May you find inspiration and solace within these pages, and may you always remember that taking care of yourself is just as important as taking care of others.

Preface

In the ever-evolving landscape of healthcare, nurses stand as unwavering pillars of support, often weathering the storms of emotional and physical demands that come with the profession. Yet, amid the chaos, the critical need for self-care is frequently overlooked. *The Self-Care Lighthouse: A Nurse's Guide to Weathering Life's Storms* was born from this realization—a call to action for nurses to prioritize their own well-being while continuing to care for others.

This guide serves as both a beacon and a sanctuary for nurses navigating the turbulent seas of their careers and personal lives. Through the pages that follow, you will discover practical strategies, insightful reflections, and the essential tools needed to cultivate resilience and maintain a balanced life. From managing stress and avoiding burnout to embracing mindfulness and fostering connections, this book offers a comprehensive approach to self-care that recognizes the unique challenges faced by those in the nursing profession.

As a nurse myself, I understand the intense pressures and emotional toll that can arise from caring for others. I have experienced firsthand the moments when the weight of the world feels overwhelming, and self-care becomes a distant thought. It is my hope that this guide will provide you with the guidance and encouragement to prioritize your own health and well-being, so you can continue to shine brightly for those you serve.

Throughout this journey, I invite you to reflect on your own experiences, to share your struggles and triumphs, and to embrace the importance of self-compassion. Just as a lighthouse guides ships through the storm, may this book illuminate your path toward a healthier, more fulfilling nursing career.

Thank you for allowing me to accompany you on this journey. Together, let us navigate the storms and emerge stronger, more resilient, and ready to embrace the light of self-care.

Table of Contents

Introduction

It is widely understood that nurses as healthcare professionals are right on the front lines attending to patients during some of the most vulnerable and stressful events of their lives. Whether it is a shift in the ER, a day on the hospital floor, or a night of call, nurses demonstrate great commitment to their patients all the time. However, in the midst of providing exceptional care, there's one important person often left out of the equation: ourselves.

This ebook is a light-hearted and easily accessible guide to self-care for nurses. Our goal is to focus on the issues of burnout, stress, and the emotional aspect of this job. You find yourself working through lunch breaks and collapsing over the keyboard by midnight believing that it is just part of the job. However, imagine if you learned that by taking even much better care of yourself—especially your mental health—you will turn out to help your patients much more?

With this fun and informative book, we want to help you remember that taking care of yourself is not a luxury but a necessity. From how to cope with stress at work to funny stories about the everyday realities of nursing, this ebook is meant to inspire, motivate, and remind you that you also deserve to have a healthy and happy life.

So, take your coffee or tea if you prefer it, put your weary legs up, and let me introduce you to the topic of self-care for nurses. And after all, you dedicate a lot of time for others and their needs – now it is time to focus on you.

Chapter 1

Mental Health - The life vest in rough seas

People sometimes find life to be like a sea; more often than not, the smooth water is overtaken by choppy waters. Impart takes of chores at work, particularly, in settings such as the health care system, there are times when the trend of stress, anxiety, and tiredness consumes one as a result of the pressures exerted. Mental health preservation turns from a value to a vital need, as putting on a life jacket in turbulent waters. Without it, we are likely to be overwhelmed by the pressures that come with life. In this section, we'll define what mental health is and offer realistic and realistic tips for keeping our minds healthy. As the author Anne Lamott said it, "Almost everything will work again if you unplug it for a few minutes, including you." This chapter is about how to learn how to "turn off" so that we can be ready to face the seas of life again with strength and vision.

Understanding Mental Health as a Healthcare Worker

However, there is a need to define why mental health is so important, particularly for the healthcare staff members. Nurses, doctors and other health care staff are under certain specific stressors. You're always supporting—patients who could be suffering from severe diseases, families under stress, or co-workers under pressure. This constant pressure can easily drain one's emotional energy, and lead to stress, anxiety, or depression.

Mental health is not just the lack of mental disorders. It's all about being able to cope with pressures of daily living, cope with stress, be a social animal, and have a reason to live. Without it, all work seems more burdensome, all choices more difficult, and all days more challenging. Mental health does not equal to not working and not being productive; it means being productive while being mentally fit to do so.

The Life Vest Analogy: Why Mental Health is Like a Life Vest

Suppose you are in the middle of the ocean and a storm starts. The sea is storming, the wind is blowing, your ship is sinking. Now imagine how you will be able to navigate the ship without a life vest. You are struggling to survive, but when you are alone, you get tired quickly, and you may be overwhelmed.

That is the reality of going through life's hurdles without giving your mental health the attention it deserves. Life vest means the behaviour patterns and strategies that let you stay on water when the strain arises as well as it provides ability to stand the test. Stress from work, stress from personal life, stress from any other form of pressure is always there but mental health is your life vest; it helps you float even in the stormy waters.

Unplugging from the Chaos: The Importance of Rest and Recovery

Perhaps one of the most effective metaphors for mental health is the statement of Anne Lamott that 'everything works better when you take it apart for a while.' As with a phone or a computer, we can get to a point where we just shut down and can no longer perform as we are overworked. Being connected all the time to the needs of our work, our children, or other obligations will at some point exhaust us and render us ineffective.

Sleep is one of the most important aspects of one's mental well-being as is the ability to relax. This doesn't just mean getting enough sleep (which is important in its own right). It's about understanding how to step back and take a mental break at various points in your day and your week.

These are those instances where you let your mind off the hook, where you do not have to worry about stress.

Practical Ways to Unplug:

- **Mindful Breathing:** If you are stressed, spend several minutes on your breathing. Breathe in for four seconds, hold the breath for four seconds, and exhale for four seconds with your eyes closed. Continue with this cycle several times. This simple act can help to regulate your nervous system and decrease stress hormones in your body.

- **Take Breaks:** Regardless of how hectic your shift is, try and take a break mid shift for at least five minutes. Take a walk, sit in the fresh air or just listen to some quiet music. These small breaks can help you to avoid the state of burnout and be more productive during work.

- **Unplug from Technology:** In the contemporary society, we are always in touch – text messages, emails, social networks, news can fill our heads with information. A good practice is to learn to put away all screens and electronic devices at least a half an hour before bedtime. Allow your brain to be idle and free from technology and any other distractions that usual occupies it.

- **Sleep Hygiene:** Sleep is not only the body's rest but the mind as well. To help you have a good night's sleep, create a night time schedule that prepares your mind and body for rest. Mornings should not have caffeine, bedroom should be cool and dark, and everyone should sleep at the same time.

Building Resilience: Your Toolkit for Mental Health

Mental health is not just about managing stress but about preparing for it, so you are ready for anything that comes your way. That is exactly what resilience means, the ability to work even when stress and anxiety levels rise and even after getting through a difficult phase. Here are key strategies to build resilience and protect your mental health:

Self-Awareness: Knowing When You Need a Life Vest

The first way to protect your mental health is to be aware of when you are beginning to have issues. Self-awareness permits the state to supervise your emotional status, and Step in before the situation worsens. Spend five minutes every day reflecting on yourself. Are you feeling overwhelmed? Exhausted? Irritable? These may be signs of burn out or stress. Please don't ignore them. If you feel overwhelmed by anger, for example, accept that feeling and then try to do something to change that before it becomes a problem.

1. Positive Relationships: *The Support Network That Helps You Stay Afloat*
As life jackets assist in floating you on water strong positive relationship can float you on water emotionally during difficult period. Be with friends who encourage you, listen to you when you want to complain, and those who know your problems. Laia on laten äästä sen näkökulma, joista tärkeää on muistaa, että ei ole yksin.
But always bear in mind, that relationships are mutual and not one-sided. Pay attention to your

relationships—call your friends, remember to ask about family, and spend time talking to people most dear to you. Such relationships do more than offer support but may also include a little happiness and companionship that help individuals mentally.

2. Mindfulness and Meditation: *Finding Your Anchor in the Present*

Mindfulness is a practice where you are being told to focus on the present moment. Life becomes so complicated and it is very easy to get stuck in the future or even in the past. Mindfulness involves deliberately paying attention to moments in one's life and actually accepting them for what they are.

You should try to practice mindfulness in your everyday life, it can be through using an app, through mindful eating or even just focusing on your breathing. Prayer or meditation for instance for just ten minutes a day has been shown to lower anxiety levels, enhance focus and bring about relaxation.

3. Exercise: *Exercise, as the Key to a Higher Level of Thinking*

Exercise is not only healthy for the physical self but also for the mental self as well. Exercise makes the body release endorphins which are chemicals in the brain that help to improve your mood. Whether it is a walk, a yoga class, or a session at the gym, the body needs to move to reduce stress, sleep better, and feel good.

Make sure that out of all the activities that you do in a week or a day, there is one that you love doing. It doesn't have to be an intense workout; even simple things like stretching or a casual walk can work wonders on your mental health.

4. Setting Boundaries: *Protecting Your Mental Space*
It is always challenging for any healthcare professional to say no. You are a caregiver and always expect to be one; you feel guilty when you prioritize yourself. However, establishing good boundaries is one of the best things that you can do for your mental health.

Understand when you are overloading yourself with work, be it the extra hours at work, more responsibilities, or other people's problems. It is acceptable to take a pause and tell yourself, "I can't take it anymore." It does not mean you are a cold-hearted person when you set your boundaries because it helps you to have energy to give when it is needed most.

5. The Power of Humor: *Laughing Through the Storm*
Last but not the least; the humor is one of the best things with which you can safeguard your mental health. Humor is the best medicine, or at least it can make life easier, especially when working in a

stressful field such as healthcare. Laughter has been known to help decrease stress, lower blood pressure and even improve the function of the immune system. Not surprisingly, humor is probably one of the best medicines one could ever want.

Laugh everyday even if that means telling a joke to a colleague or watching a comedian on television at night. Learn to laugh at life—because in the middle of a storm, a smile is the rope that can save your life.

Speaking of which, your mental health is your life jacket when you find yourself in the middle of the ocean of life. When you are able to disconnect, rebound, foster relationships that are meaningful, and enjoy laughter, you can preserve your head health, and help those you consider important with fresh energy. Just to repeat, self-care is not something you do when you have spare time, but the necessity to become successful both at work and at home.

Chapter 2

Self-Care - The Lifeboat Emotional Rescue

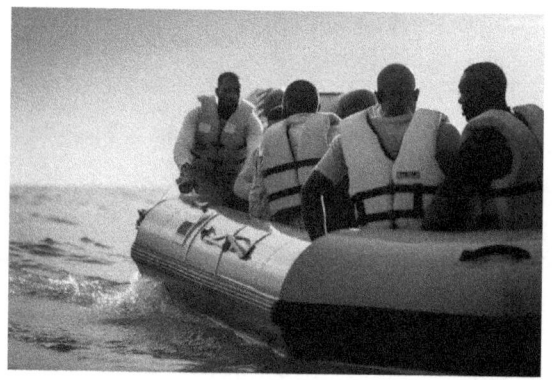

Lost at sea of life where stress and responsibilities engulf like ocean waves on a stormy day self-care becomes our only lifeline – a lifeline to one's soul. We can easily neglect ourselves while performing our duties, not to mention those of us who are in the caregiving line of work. Nonetheless, taking care of oneself is not a self-indulgence; it is a survival and living tactic which should be embraced.

Understanding Self-Care: More Than Just a Buzzword

Self-care can be misinterpreted as some new thing or a mere fad or even referred to as the act of being lazy or self-serving. Actually it is a combination of activities aimed at sustaining and promoting human health physically, emotionally and mentally. Self care does not mean purchasing occasional extras; it means making better decisions that improve our health.

Self-care should be seen as the life buoy that is thrown to you when you are flailing in the water that is choppy. For instance, just as one may look forward to the lifeboat during a storm for safety and stability so can or self-care practices in the 'emotional storm' shaping our daily existence.

The Importance of Self-Care

Preventing Burnout

For the employees who work in stressful occupations like healthcare or education, burnout is a real possibility. It results in physical, emotional and mental fatigue reducing your ability to attend to the needs of others. Self-care helps to reduce this risk because it gives you the means to replenish your energy. They mean that by making yourself whole, you become more able to take care of others without jeopardizing your own health.

Enhancing Mental Health

Practices of self-care are a direct predictor of better mental health. Mindfulness, exercise or time spent with family and friends could greatly help or fully eliminate stress, anxiety and depression. They also contribute to the provision of uniqueness, hence a balance as well as order in enhancing emotional regulation. Taking care of yourself is easy and helps to have positive thoughts to handle the struggles of life.

Healthy relationships

When you are taking care of yourself, then you are in a better position to take care of your relationships. Caring for your needs helps you to be more responsive to the people you love. When you are emotionally healthier, your relationships with other people can be more satisfying and real. Also, seeing the specifics of self-care is an effective way to encourage people to show the same concern about their own health.

Increasing Productivity

Taking care of oneself can help improve on productivity as a result of the investment made. If you take time off work, you come back with a fresh attitude and are ready to tackle the job at hand. This can mean work productivity improvement, increased creativity and an enhanced potential for problem solving.

Practical Self-Care Strategies: Setting Sail on Your Lifeboat

That is why it is crucial to know how to start the process of self-care, and below, you will find some tips to begin with. Remember, that there is no universally correct way of handling it, everyone is different and can have different reactions to the same stimulus. The idea is to discover what matters to you and to focus on it.

Establish a Routine

Making a schedule for self-care is useful because it allows time to be set aside in the middle of the countless tasks. One way could be to plan what activities are going to be used to self care for the week and then carve out particular segments of the day for the respective activity. This could be a walk, reading, genital or other kind of meditation or any other form of creative pastime. It is important to be regular, the more often you practice self-care, the more it will become a habit.

Practice Mindfulness

Mindfulness often pertains to paying attention to the current occurrence and this can help as a self care tool. Fermented foods can ease anxiety and curb other negative feelings so they have a way of affecting the mood. Use mindfulness methods like meditation or probably taking deep breath, get affirmative-minded tricks into your lifestyle. As little as five minutes spent on deep breathing can help reduce stress and change your mood.

Engage in Physical Activity

Exercise is one of the most important components of personal care. It makes you stronger physically but also leaves you with good hormones known as endorphins that make you feel happy. Choose an exercise that you like, it can be walking, dancing, yoga, or playing sports. Try to get at least 30 minutes of exercise a couple of times per week this will definitely improve your mood and energy.

Prioritize Sleep

Sound sleep is essential to the health of the emotions as well as the physical body. If we are well-rested then we can be able to reason better, make good decisions and even manage stress. It is important for a child to practice a good night's sleep, have a good sleep environment, and should sleep for 7 to 9 hours every night. Getting adequate sleep is one of the most effective self-care actions and yet often the most neglected.

Nourish Your Body
The food that we take affects our mood and energy levels in a great way. Try to consume foods that are low in calories, high in fiber, vitamins and minerals, and lean meats. Pay attention to what you eat and attempt to eat without distractions. This activity can be also a method of transformed care for the body; try new recipes and pamper yourself with tasty and healthy dishes.

Connect with Nature

The literature review indicates that time spent in nature decreases stress and increases mood. It's important that you take time to go for a walk in the park, hiking or just sit in your green area even if it's mini garden. Moreso, nature has a marvelous way of meeting us at our human level and can be relied upon to bring about our rejuvenation.

Engage in Creative Activities

One can find that creativity can be a great way to deal with stress. Do things that can help you to be creative, this may include painting, writing, gardening or doing some form of crafting. This might be a sense of achievement and enjoyment once you permit your creativity to flow freeing oneself from work related stress.

Overcoming Barriers to Self-Care

Despite the clear benefits of self-care, many people struggle to prioritize it. Here are some common barriers and how to overcome them:

Time Constraints

It's easy to feel like there's not enough time in the day for self-care. To address this, start small. Even dedicating just five or ten minutes a day to a self-care practice can make a difference. Gradually increase the time as it becomes a more integral part of your routine.

Guilt

Many caregivers feel guilty about taking time for themselves. It's essential to reframe this mindset; self-care is not selfish. When you take care of your own needs, you are better equipped to care for others. Remind yourself that prioritizing your well-being ultimately benefits everyone around you.

Unrealistic Expectations

Some may think self-care needs to be extravagant to be effective. In reality, self-care can be as simple as enjoying a hot cup of tea or taking a short walk. Focus on finding activities that resonate with you and fit your lifestyle.

The Ripple Effect of Self-Care

Prioritizing self-care has a ripple effect on your life and the lives of those around you. When you engage in regular self-care, you:

- **Improve Your Relationships**: As you nurture your emotional well-being, you become more present and attentive in your interactions with loved ones.

- **Enhance Your Work Performance**: A balanced and refreshed mind translates into increased productivity, creativity, and effectiveness in your job.
- **Inspire Others**: By modeling self-care behaviors, you encourage friends, family, and colleagues to prioritize their well-being, creating a culture of care and support.

Self-care is your lifeboat in the turbulent seas of life—a necessary strategy for emotional rescue. It empowers you to prioritize your well-being, build resilience, and navigate challenges with grace. By establishing a self-care routine that resonates with you, you're taking essential steps towards better mental, emotional, and physical health.

Chapter 3

Building Resilience - The Captain Of Your Ship

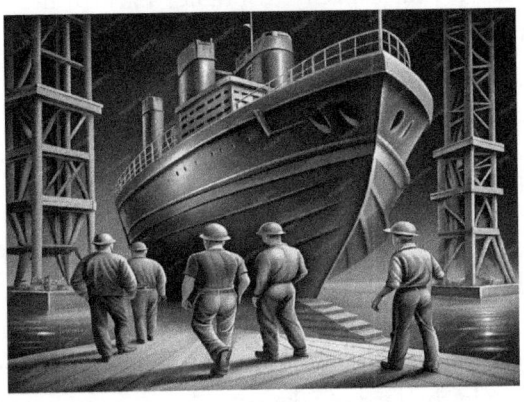

In the turbulent seas of life, building resilience is like taking the helm of your ship. Resilience equips you with the skills to navigate through adversity, enabling you to withstand the storms that life throws your way. Just as a skilled captain relies on their knowledge and instincts to steer their vessel, developing resilience allows you to harness your inner strength and humor to confront challenges head-on. As author Nora Ephron reminds us, "Above all, be the heroine of your life, not the victim."

This mindset shift is crucial: instead of feeling overwhelmed by circumstances, resilience empowers you to reclaim control over your life's narrative. In this chapter, we'll explore what resilience truly means, the importance of humor in building resilience, and practical strategies to enhance your capacity to bounce back from life's challenges.

Understanding Resilience

What Is Resilience?
Resilience is often defined as the ability to bounce back from setbacks, adapt to change, and keep going in the face of adversity. It's not about being unaffected by challenges; rather, it's about developing the mental and emotional strength to manage them effectively. Resilience enables you to face difficulties with courage, determination, and a proactive approach.

The Importance of Resilience
Resilience is crucial for several reasons:

- **Emotional Well-Being**: Resilient individuals tend to experience lower levels of stress, anxiety, and depression. They are better equipped to handle life's challenges and maintain a positive outlook.
- **Enhanced Problem-Solving Skills**: Resilience fosters adaptability, allowing you to approach problems with creativity and flexibility. You become more open to finding solutions rather than feeling stuck.
- **Stronger Relationships**: Resilient people often build stronger social connections. They are better able to communicate their needs and seek support, which enhances their interpersonal relationships.
- **Greater Life Satisfaction**: By cultivating resilience, you can navigate life's ups and downs with grace, leading to a more fulfilling and satisfying life experience.

The Role of Humor in Resilience

Humor plays a vital role in building resilience. It serves as a coping mechanism that can lighten the weight of difficult situations. Here's how humor contributes to resilience:

Perspective Shift

Humor allows you to reframe challenging situations, helping you to see them from a different angle. Instead of feeling defeated by adversity, laughter can provide a fresh perspective, making it easier to cope with stress and find solutions.

Emotional Release

Laughter serves as an emotional release, reducing tension and promoting feelings of joy and connection. It helps alleviate stress and anxiety, creating a buffer against the emotional turmoil that challenges can bring.

Strengthening Connections

Sharing a laugh with others fosters a sense of camaraderie and strengthens relationships. Humor helps build bonds with friends, family, and colleagues, creating a support network that is essential for resilience.

Practical Strategies to Build Resilience

Building resilience is a lifelong process that requires intentional effort. Here are some practical strategies to help you develop your capacity for resilience and steer your ship with confidence:

Cultivate a Growth Mindset

A growth mindset is the belief that you can develop your abilities and intelligence through effort and learning. Embrace challenges as opportunities for growth rather than viewing them as threats. This mindset shift can enhance your resilience, allowing you to approach difficulties with curiosity and determination.

Establish a Support Network

Building and maintaining a strong support network is crucial for resilience. Surround yourself with positive, supportive people who uplift you during difficult times. Seek out friendships and relationships that encourage open communication, empathy, and mutual support.

Practice Self-Compassion

Being kind to yourself is a key aspect of resilience. Recognize that it's okay to feel vulnerable or struggle at times. Practice self-compassion by treating yourself with the same kindness and understanding that you would offer a friend facing similar challenges.

Develop Problem-Solving Skills

Resilience involves effective problem-solving. When faced with a challenge, break it down into manageable steps. Identify potential solutions, evaluate their pros and cons, and take action. This proactive approach empowers you to tackle obstacles with confidence.

Embrace Change

Change is an inevitable part of life, and embracing it can enhance your resilience. Rather than resisting change, practice flexibility and adaptability. Learn to see change as an opportunity for growth and new experiences.

Prioritize Self-Care

Taking care of your physical, emotional, and mental well-being is fundamental to building resilience. Prioritize self-care activities that recharge your batteries, such as exercise, mindfulness practices, and engaging in hobbies that bring you joy.

Set Realistic Goals

Establishing realistic goals can provide a sense of purpose and direction, helping you stay focused during challenging times. Break larger goals into smaller, achievable steps to maintain motivation and track progress.

Reflect and Learn

After facing a challenging situation, take time to reflect on the experience. What did you learn about yourself? What coping strategies worked well? Reflecting on your experiences can help you build resilience for the future.

Navigating Life's Storms

As you develop your resilience, remember that challenges are an inherent part of life's journey. Each storm you face can serve as an opportunity to strengthen your inner captain—the part of you that steers your ship with confidence and determination.

When adversity strikes, consider how you can apply your resilience strategies:

- **Stay Calm**: In turbulent times, maintain your composure. Take a deep breath, assess the situation, and remember your coping strategies.

- **Use Humor**: When appropriate, find the humor in the situation. Sharing a laugh can lighten the mood and provide a fresh perspective.

- **Seek Support**: Don't hesitate to reach out to your support network. Lean on friends and family for encouragement, advice, or simply a listening ear.

- **Reframe Challenges**: Shift your mindset to see challenges as opportunities for growth. Ask yourself what you can learn from the situation and how it can contribute to your resilience.

Building resilience is an ongoing journey—one that requires intention and effort. As the captain of your ship, you have the power to navigate life's storms with grace and confidence. By cultivating resilience, embracing humor, and employing practical strategies, you can steer your vessel through choppy waters and emerge stronger on the other side.

Nora Ephron's words serve as a powerful reminder that you are the heroine of your life. Rather than allowing circumstances to dictate your path, take charge and steer your ship with determination and courage. The seas may be unpredictable, but with resilience as your compass, you can navigate through the storms and chart a course towards a brighter, more fulfilling future.

Chapter 4

The Power Of Laughter - A Much-Needed Anchor

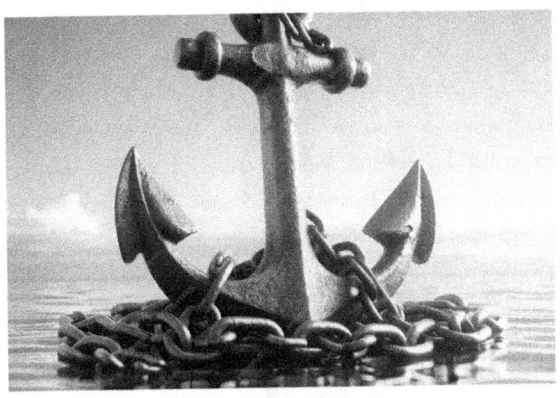

In the sea of life where everything is unpredictable and where stress and challenges are a part of day to day life, laughter are a stabilizer. According to the writer and humorist, Erma Bombeck, "If you can't make it better, you can laugh at it." This point of view emphasizes the importance of laughter in relation to changes which take place in human life. Even beyond missionaries and providers, humor is not only beneficial to individuals'emotional state but is also a therapeutic weapon and relation builder.

The Healing Power of Humor

A Natural Stress Reliever

Laughter triggers the release of endorphins, the body's natural feel-good chemicals. This physiological response reduces stress hormones, promoting an overall sense of well-being. When we laugh, our body relaxes, heart rate decreases, and tension dissipates. The act of laughing can serve as a natural antidote to stress, allowing us to cope more effectively with challenges.

Enhancing Mental Health

Humor has been shown to have significant benefits for mental health. Regular laughter can help alleviate symptoms of anxiety and depression, providing a much-needed boost to our emotional state. It creates a sense of joy and connection, which can counteract feelings of isolation and hopelessness. Humor acts as a powerful reminder that, even in difficult times, there is always something to smile about.

Strengthening Relationships

Laughter has an innate ability to bring people together. Shared humor creates bonds, fosters intimacy, and enhances social interactions. When we laugh with others, we create positive experiences that strengthen our relationships and build a sense of community. The connections formed through laughter can be invaluable, especially during challenging times when we need support and encouragement.

The Role of Humor in Everyday Life

Finding Humor in Everyday Situations

Life is full of challenges, but within those challenges lies the potential for humor. Embracing the absurdity of life's situations can transform how we cope with stress. Here are some examples of finding humor in everyday scenarios:

- **Workplace Mishaps**: Imagine a day at work where nothing seems to go right. Instead of getting frustrated, share the hilarity of the mishaps with colleagues. Turn a forgotten presentation into a funny story that leaves everyone laughing instead of groaning.

- **Parenting Fails**: Parenting is a journey filled with unexpected moments. Share the comical side of parenting, like the time your child mistook your favorite lipstick for face paint. These humorous anecdotes not only lighten the mood but also create a sense of camaraderie among parents facing similar challenges.
- **Health Scares**: Medical appointments can be nerve-wracking, but sharing humorous stories about awkward moments in the doctor's office can provide comic relief. A lighthearted approach can help demystify medical experiences and make them feel less intimidating.

Utilizing Humor as a Coping Mechanism

In difficult situations, finding humor can be a powerful coping mechanism. Here's how to incorporate humor into your coping strategies:

- **Use Comedy as an Escape**: Watching stand-up comedy, sitcoms, or funny movies can provide a much-needed escape from reality. Laughter becomes a form of self-care that allows you to detach from stressors and immerse yourself in joy.
- **Share Jokes and Anecdotes**: Engage in conversations with friends or family

members where sharing funny stories or jokes is encouraged. This can create a positive atmosphere and remind everyone of the lighter side of life.

- **Create a Laughter Ritual:** Dedicate specific times each week to laughter—whether it's hosting a comedy night at home, attending a local improv show, or joining a laughter yoga class. Establishing a routine focused on laughter reinforces its importance in your life.

Stories That Will Leave You in Stitches

To illustrate the healing power of laughter, let's share a few lighthearted stories that capture the essence of humor in our lives.

The Grocery Store Mix-Up

A friend once shared a hilarious experience she had while grocery shopping. She was in a rush, trying to grab ingredients for a dinner party. As she hurried through the aisles, she picked up what she thought was chicken breast but later discovered it was tofu.

Later that evening, while preparing the meal, her guest arrived early. Not wanting to seem disorganized, she decided to play it off. When her friend asked about the dish, she confidently stated, "I'm trying out a new recipe—chicken à la surprise!" The look on her friend's face when they both took a bite was priceless, and they spent the evening laughing over her culinary mishap.

The Technology Fiasco

In our tech-driven world, it's easy to feel overwhelmed by gadgets. One day, a coworker was trying to present a project using a new software application. As she navigated the program, she accidentally shared her screen, revealing a series of cat memes she had saved for "emergency breaks."

Instead of panicking, she embraced the situation. "Well, I guess you all now know my secret to staying sane during deadlines!" She quickly turned the awkward moment into a lighthearted discussion about their favorite memes, creating a memorable bonding experience.

The Accidental Text

Picture this: a husband attempting to send a flirty text to his wife, but accidentally sending it to his boss instead. The text read, "Can't wait to see you tonight; I'll wear the red dress!" When he realized his mistake, he immediately texted his boss to explain.

To his surprise, his boss responded with a humorous twist: "I'll bring the wine!" Instead of feeling embarrassed, the husband decided to embrace the humor of the situation, recounting the story at dinner that evening. They both ended up in fits of laughter, solidifying the idea that laughter can diffuse even the most awkward situations.

Cultivating a Culture of Laughter

In the Workplace

Creating a culture of laughter in the workplace can have significant benefits for morale and productivity. Here are some ways to cultivate this culture:

- **Encourage Humor**: Allow employees to share funny stories or memes during team meetings. Laughter can break the ice and foster a more relaxed atmosphere.

- **Celebrate Light Moments**: Recognize and celebrate moments of humor, whether it's through awards for the "funniest email" or "best joke of the week." This creates an environment where humor is valued.
- **Incorporate Playfulness**: Organize team-building activities that emphasize fun and creativity. Activities like improv workshops or comedy nights can help teams bond through laughter.

In Personal Relationships

Fostering laughter in your personal relationships can enhance connections and create cherished memories. Here's how to do it:

- **Make Time for Fun**: Schedule regular game nights or outings that emphasize fun and laughter. The more you prioritize joy, the stronger your relationships will become.
- **Be Playful**: Embrace playfulness in your interactions with loved ones. Use inside jokes, playful teasing, or silly challenges to foster an atmosphere of laughter.
- **Share Laughter**: Create a shared collection of funny videos, jokes, or stories with your loved ones. Having a go-to list of laughs can help lift spirits when times get tough.

Much of what may happen in life is turbulent, but laughter is that Ruby in the rough that holds everything together and promises calm. Recognizing that laughter can be therapeutic for your mind as well as your spirit not only benefits the individual, but serves to deepen relationships with others.

In a world that is often weights with so much burden, then laughter becomes that tiny spark that tells us that there is also happiness in struggles. If you can remake your thinking to find humor in every situation, then life becomes one big comedy when going through the hardships. Therefore, when you are out there again, chasing the waves of life, try to find the laughter that is going to keep you afloat – for what else does the great humorist Erma Bombeck tell us is your best bet when you cannot make things better?

Chapter 5

Conclusion - Smooth Sailing Ahead

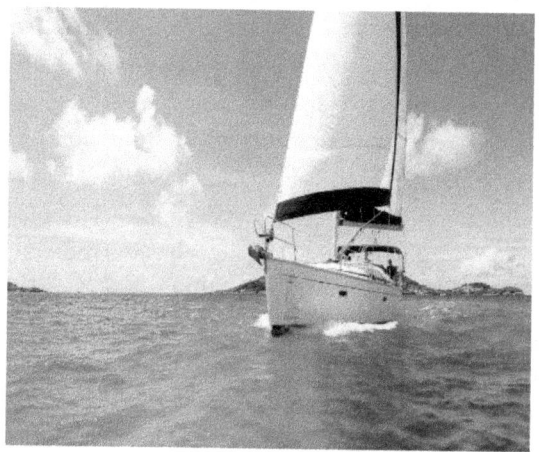

In the course of this ebook, the need to encourage self-care among nurses has been emphasized time and again. In light of daily struggles, crucial settings and stakes, and emotional pressures, it is obviating the value of, or arguing against, the need to maintain/protect one's mental health by stating that, for practitioners, doing so is merely positive or helpful to their work...; Mental health welfare is not a luxury; it is mandatory to receive and reciprocate high-quality care for and from our patients to succeed at what we do.

Author Maya Angelou's profound words resonate deeply: In life you will face so many challenges but remember you should never lose. In fact, it may be necessary to experience the defeats so that you can know who you are, what you can rise from, how you can still come out of it." But when we hear those words it helps us remember that struggle is a part of life and struggle yields with it new strengths.

The Journey of Self-Care

Embracing Self-Care as a Journey

Self-care is not a one-time event; it is a continuous journey that requires regular attention and adjustment. Just as sailors adjust their sails to harness the winds, we must adapt our self-care practices to fit our evolving needs. Whether it's developing resilience, engaging in humor, or practicing mindfulness, self-care can take many forms. Each step you take on this journey is a testament to your commitment to yourself and your profession.

The Importance of Reflection

As you navigate your self-care journey, take time to reflect on your experiences. What strategies have worked well for you? Are there areas where you could improve? Reflecting on your journey not only deepens your understanding of your needs but also reinforces the importance of self-care as a foundational aspect of your life as a healthcare professional. This reflection helps you recognize patterns and adjust your approach, ensuring that self-care remains a priority.

Creating a Self-Care Toolbox
Consider building a "self-care toolbox" filled with techniques, resources, and activities that bring you joy and relaxation. This could include practices such as meditation, exercise, hobbies, or even connecting with loved ones. Having a variety of options readily available empowers you to choose what you need in any given moment. When you encounter rough waters, you can reach into your toolbox for the right tools to guide you toward calm.

Navigating Challenges with Confidence

Facing Adversity with Courage

In our profession, we often encounter challenging situations that test our resilience and resolve. However, by prioritizing self-care, we equip ourselves to face these adversities with courage. Remember that encountering difficulties is not a reflection of failure but rather a part of our growth process. Each challenge presents an opportunity to learn more about ourselves and our capabilities.

Building a Support Network

As nurses, we are not alone on this journey. Building a strong support network—comprising colleagues, friends, and family—provides essential encouragement and understanding. Sharing experiences, both triumphs and defeats, fosters a sense of belonging and reinforces the idea that we are all navigating similar seas. A supportive network can help you weather the storms of life, reminding you that you have others to lean on during difficult times.

Letting Your Lighthouse Shine Bright

The Self-Care Lighthouse
Imagine self-care as a lighthouse, guiding you through the tumultuous seas of life. It stands as a beacon of hope, illuminating the path to calm waters. When you prioritize your mental and emotional well-being, you allow that lighthouse to shine even brighter, not just for yourself, but for your patients and those around you. By taking care of yourself, you create a ripple effect, encouraging others to prioritize their well-being as well.

Sharing Your Journey
As you embark on this self-care journey, consider sharing your experiences with others. By openly discussing the importance of self-care, you inspire your colleagues and friends to take their mental health seriously. This collective commitment to self-care fosters a culture of support and well-being within the healthcare community, leading to better outcomes for both staff and patients.

Celebrating Your Wins
Finally, celebrate your victories, no matter how small they may seem. Whether it's taking a few moments for yourself during a busy shift,

attending a self-care workshop, or successfully navigating a challenging day, each accomplishment deserves recognition. Celebrating your wins reinforces the positive impact of self-care, reminding you that every step taken is a step toward a healthier, more balanced life.

Smooth Sailing Ahead

As a final note, the general idea is that excellent crisis management is not about doing the mishap prevention but about handling these situations with grace and vigor for the storm to come. Neglecting self is something that is not for careless people but for every nurse who wants to deliver the best health care services. If you understand yourself better, appreciate the healing power of laughter and have support in your workplace, you can build a personal and professional life with a wonderful balance.

In this book, the self-care lighthouse will help you find your bearings and show the way forward when the going gets rough. May you find happiness, relationships, and courage in the process to everything you decided to do for yourself. To the future: clear waters wait ahead – so it's time to get ready for the voyage!

References in APA Format

1. Lamott, A. (1995). Bird by bird: Some instructions on writing and life. Anchor.
2. Ephron, N. (2006). I feel bad about my neck: And other thoughts on being a woman. Alfred A. Knopf.
3. Bombeck, E. (1979). *Aunt Erma's cope book*. McGraw-Hill.
4. Angelou, M. (1990). *I shall not be moved*. Bantam Books.

In-Text Citations for Each Quote

1. "Almost everything will work again if you unplug it for a few minutes, including you." (Lamott, 1995, p. 28)

Relevance: This quote emphasizes the importance of taking breaks and practicing self-care. In the context of nursing, where the demands can be relentless, it serves as a reminder that stepping back can lead to rejuvenation and improved mental health.

2. "Above all, be the heroine of your life, not the victim." (Ephron, 2006, p. 17)

Relevance: Ephron's quote encourages empowerment and resilience. It highlights the need for nurses to take charge of their narratives and prioritize their well-being, reinforcing the theme of building resilience as a fundamental aspect of self-care.

3. "If you can't make it better, you can laugh at it." (Bombeck, 1979, p. 81)

Relevance: This quote speaks to the healing power of humor in coping with life's challenges. In nursing, where stress is prevalent, the ability to find humor in difficult situations can foster camaraderie and support, reminding healthcare professionals that laughter can be a valuable coping mechanism.

4. "You may encounter many defeats, but you must not be defeated. In fact, it may be necessary to encounter the defeats, so you can know who you are, what you can rise from, how you can still come out of it." (Angelou, 1990, p. 117)

Relevance: Angelou's quote encapsulates the essence of resilience. It acknowledges that setbacks are part of the journey and encourages nurses to learn from their experiences. This aligns with the overarching message of the ebook: that prioritizing self-care and resilience ultimately leads to personal and professional growth.